My Food Allergy Journal

If Lost, Return To:

_____

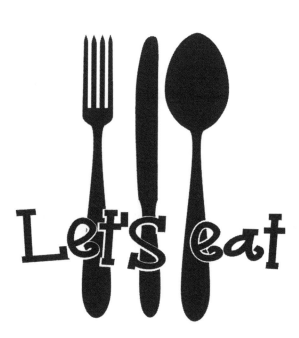

Date:————————————

Breakfast Time:	Symptoms/Reactions

Lunch Time:	Symptoms/Reactions

Dinner Time:	Symptoms/Reactions

Water Intake:

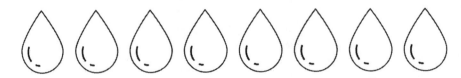

Snack 1	Time:	Symptoms/Reactions

Snack 1	Time:	Symptoms/Reactions

Snack 1	Time:	Symptoms/Reactions

Notes:

Date:_____

Breakfast Time:	Symptoms/Reactions

Lunch Time:	Symptoms/Reactions

Dinner Time:	Symptoms/Reactions

Water Intake:

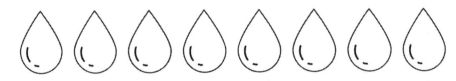

Snack 1 Time:	Symptoms/Reactions

Snack 1 Time:	Symptoms/Reactions

Snack 1 Time:	Symptoms/Reactions

Notes:

_____

_____

_____

_____

_____

Date:_____

Breakfast Time:	Symptoms/Reactions

Lunch Time:	Symptoms/Reactions

Dinner Time:	Symptoms/Reactions

Water Intake:

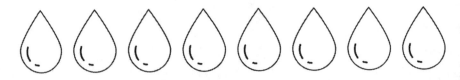

Snack 1 Time:	Symptoms/Reactions

Snack 1 Time:	Symptoms/Reactions

Snack 1 Time:	Symptoms/Reactions

Notes:

_____

_____

_____

_____

_____

_____

Date:_____

Breakfast	Time:	Symptoms/Reactions

Lunch	Time:	Symptoms/Reactions

Dinner	Time:	Symptoms/Reactions

Water Intake:

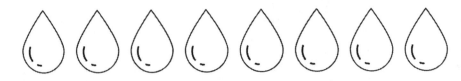

Snack 1 Time:	Symptoms/Reactions

Snack 1 Time:	Symptoms/Reactions

Snack 1 Time:	Symptoms/Reactions

Notes:

_____

_____

_____

_____

_____

Date:_____

Breakfast	Time:	Symptoms/Reactions

Lunch	Time:	Symptoms/Reactions

Dinner	Time:	Symptoms/Reactions

Water Intake:

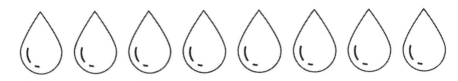

Snack 1	Time:	Symptoms/Reactions

Snack 1	Time:	Symptoms/Reactions

Snack 1	Time:	Symptoms/Reactions

Notes:

_____

_____

_____

_____

_____

Date:_____

Breakfast Time:	Symptoms/Reactions

Lunch Time:	Symptoms/Reactions

Dinner Time:	Symptoms/Reactions

Water Intake:

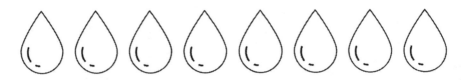

Snack 1 Time:	Symptoms/Reactions

Snack 1 Time:	Symptoms/Reactions

Snack 1 Time:	Symptoms/Reactions

Notes:

Date:_____

Breakfast	Time:	Symptoms/Reactions

Lunch	Time:	Symptoms/Reactions

Dinner	Time:	Symptoms/Reactions

Water Intake:

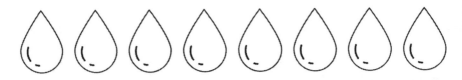

Snack 1 Time:	Symptoms/Reactions

Snack 1 Time:	Symptoms/Reactions

Snack 1 Time:	Symptoms/Reactions

Notes:

Date:_____

Breakfast Time:	Symptoms/Reactions

Lunch Time:	Symptoms/Reactions

Dinner Time:	Symptoms/Reactions

Water Intake:

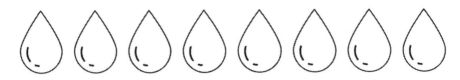

Snack 1 Time:	Symptoms/Reactions

Snack 1 Time:	Symptoms/Reactions

Snack 1 Time:	Symptoms/Reactions

Notes:

_____

_____

_____

_____

_____

_____

Date:_____

Breakfast Time:	Symptoms/Reactions

Lunch Time:	Symptoms/Reactions

Dinner Time:	Symptoms/Reactions

Water Intake:

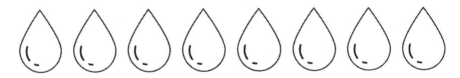

Snack 1 Time:	Symptoms/Reactions

Snack 1 Time:	Symptoms/Reactions

Snack 1 Time:	Symptoms/Reactions

Notes:

Date:_____

Breakfast Time:	Symptoms/Reactions

Lunch Time:	Symptoms/Reactions

Dinner Time:	Symptoms/Reactions

Water Intake:

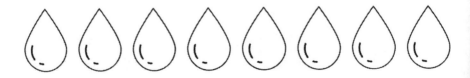

Snack 1 Time:	Symptoms/Reactions

Snack 1 Time:	Symptoms/Reactions

Snack 1 Time:	Symptoms/Reactions

Notes:

Date:_____

Breakfast Time:	Symptoms/Reactions

Lunch Time:	Symptoms/Reactions

Dinner Time:	Symptoms/Reactions

Water Intake:

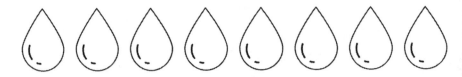

Snack 1 Time:	Symptoms/Reactions

Snack 1 Time:	Symptoms/Reactions

Snack 1 Time:	Symptoms/Reactions

Notes:

Date:_____

Breakfast Time:	Symptoms/Reactions

Lunch Time:	Symptoms/Reactions

Dinner Time:	Symptoms/Reactions

Water Intake:

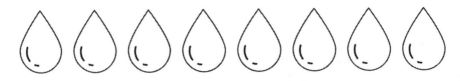

Snack 1 Time:	Symptoms/Reactions

Snack 1 Time:	Symptoms/Reactions

Snack 1 Time:	Symptoms/Reactions

Notes:

Date:_____

Breakfast Time:	Symptoms/Reactions

Lunch Time:	Symptoms/Reactions

Dinner Time:	Symptoms/Reactions

Water Intake:

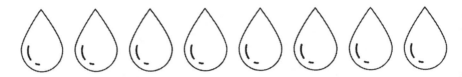

Snack 1 Time:	Symptoms/Reactions

Snack 1 Time:	Symptoms/Reactions

Snack 1 Time:	Symptoms/Reactions

Notes:

Date:———————————————

Breakfast Time:	Symptoms/Reactions

Lunch Time:	Symptoms/Reactions

Dinner Time:	Symptoms/Reactions

Water Intake:

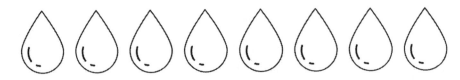

Snack 1	Time:	Symptoms/Reactions

Snack 1	Time:	Symptoms/Reactions

Snack 1	Time:	Symptoms/Reactions

Notes:

Date:_____

Breakfast	Time:	Symptoms/Reactions

Lunch	Time:	Symptoms/Reactions

Dinner	Time:	Symptoms/Reactions

Water Intake:

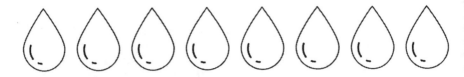

Snack 1 Time:	Symptoms/Reactions

Snack 1 Time:	Symptoms/Reactions

Snack 1 Time:	Symptoms/Reactions

Notes:

Date:_____

Breakfast Time:	Symptoms/Reactions

Lunch Time:	Symptoms/Reactions

Dinner Time:	Symptoms/Reactions

Water Intake:

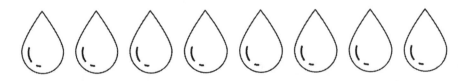

Snack 1 Time:	Symptoms/Reactions

Snack 1 Time:	Symptoms/Reactions

Snack 1 Time:	Symptoms/Reactions

Notes:

_____

_____

_____

_____

_____

Date:_____

Breakfast	Time:	Symptoms/Reactions

Lunch	Time:	Symptoms/Reactions

Dinner	Time:	Symptoms/Reactions

Water Intake:

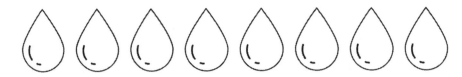

Snack 1 Time:	Symptoms/Reactions

Snack 1 Time:	Symptoms/Reactions

Snack 1 Time:	Symptoms/Reactions

Notes:

_____

_____

_____

_____

_____

Date:_____

Breakfast	Time:	Symptoms/Reactions

Lunch	Time:	Symptoms/Reactions

Dinner	Time:	Symptoms/Reactions

Water Intake:

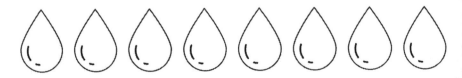

Snack 1 Time:	Symptoms/Reactions

Snack 1 Time:	Symptoms/Reactions

Snack 1 Time:	Symptoms/Reactions

Notes:

Date:_____

Breakfast	Time:	Symptoms/Reactions

Lunch	Time:	Symptoms/Reactions

Dinner	Time:	Symptoms/Reactions

Water Intake:

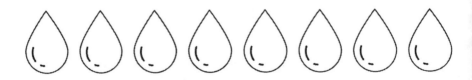

Snack 1	Time:	Symptoms/Reactions

Snack 1	Time:	Symptoms/Reactions

Snack 1	Time:	Symptoms/Reactions

Notes:

Date:_____

Breakfast	Time:	Symptoms/Reactions

Lunch	Time:	Symptoms/Reactions

Dinner	Time:	Symptoms/Reactions

Water Intake:

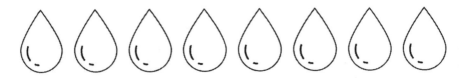

Snack 1 Time:	Symptoms/Reactions

Snack 1 Time:	Symptoms/Reactions

Snack 1 Time:	Symptoms/Reactions

Notes:

Date:_____

Breakfast	Time:	Symptoms/Reactions

Lunch	Time:	Symptoms/Reactions

Dinner	Time:	Symptoms/Reactions

Water Intake:

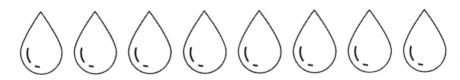

Snack 1 Time:	Symptoms/Reactions

Snack 1 Time:	Symptoms/Reactions

Snack 1 Time:	Symptoms/Reactions

Notes:

Date:_____

Breakfast	Time:	Symptoms/Reactions

Lunch	Time:	Symptoms/Reactions

Dinner	Time:	Symptoms/Reactions

Water Intake:

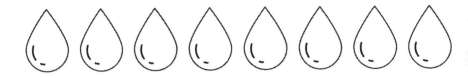

Snack 1 Time:	Symptoms/Reactions

Snack 1 Time:	Symptoms/Reactions

Snack 1 Time:	Symptoms/Reactions

Notes:

Date:_____

Breakfast Time:	Symptoms/Reactions

Lunch Time:	Symptoms/Reactions

Dinner Time:	Symptoms/Reactions

Water Intake:

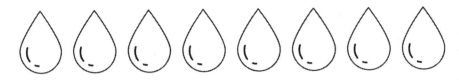

Snack 1 Time:	Symptoms/Reactions

Snack 1 Time:	Symptoms/Reactions

Snack 1 Time:	Symptoms/Reactions

Notes:

_____

_____

_____

_____

_____

Date:_____

Breakfast Time:	Symptoms/Reactions

Lunch Time:	Symptoms/Reactions

Dinner Time:	Symptoms/Reactions

Water Intake:

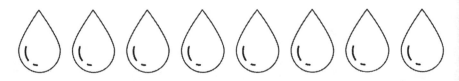

Snack 1 Time:	Symptoms/Reactions

Snack 1 Time:	Symptoms/Reactions

Snack 1 Time:	Symptoms/Reactions

Notes:

Date:_____

Breakfast	Time:	Symptoms/Reactions

Lunch	Time:	Symptoms/Reactions

Dinner	Time:	Symptoms/Reactions

Water Intake:

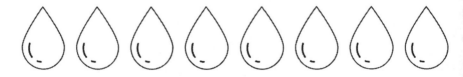

Snack 1 Time:	Symptoms/Reactions

Snack 1 Time:	Symptoms/Reactions

Snack 1 Time:	Symptoms/Reactions

Notes:

Date:_____

Breakfast Time:	Symptoms/Reactions

Lunch Time:	Symptoms/Reactions

Dinner Time:	Symptoms/Reactions

Water Intake:

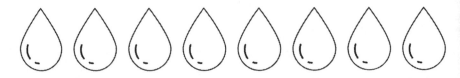

Snack 1 Time:	Symptoms/Reactions

Snack 1 Time:	Symptoms/Reactions

Snack 1 Time:	Symptoms/Reactions

Notes:

_____

_____

_____

_____

_____

Date:_____

Breakfast Time:	Symptoms/Reactions

Lunch Time:	Symptoms/Reactions

Dinner Time:	Symptoms/Reactions

Water Intake:

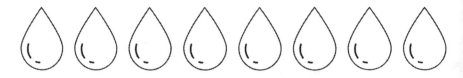

Snack 1 Time:	Symptoms/Reactions

Snack 1 Time:	Symptoms/Reactions

Snack 1 Time:	Symptoms/Reactions

Notes:

Date:_____

Breakfast Time:	Symptoms/Reactions

Lunch Time:	Symptoms/Reactions

Dinner Time:	Symptoms/Reactions

Water Intake:

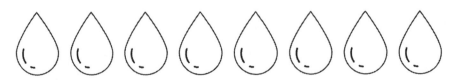

Snack 1 Time:	Symptoms/Reactions

Snack 1 Time:	Symptoms/Reactions

Snack 1 Time:	Symptoms/Reactions

Notes:

Date:_____

Breakfast	Time:	Symptoms/Reactions

Lunch	Time:	Symptoms/Reactions

Dinner	Time:	Symptoms/Reactions

Water Intake:

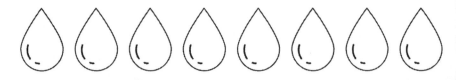

Snack 1 Time:	Symptoms/Reactions

Snack 1 Time:	Symptoms/Reactions

Snack 1 Time:	Symptoms/Reactions

Notes:

_____

_____

_____

_____

_____

Date:_____

Breakfast Time:	Symptoms/Reactions

Lunch Time:	Symptoms/Reactions

Dinner Time:	Symptoms/Reactions

Water Intake:

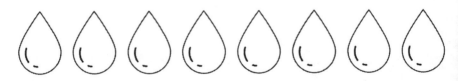

Snack 1	Time:	Symptoms/Reactions

Snack 1	Time:	Symptoms/Reactions

Snack 1	Time:	Symptoms/Reactions

Notes:

_____

_____

_____

_____

_____

Date:_____

Breakfast Time:	Symptoms/Reactions

Lunch Time:	Symptoms/Reactions

Dinner Time:	Symptoms/Reactions

Water Intake:

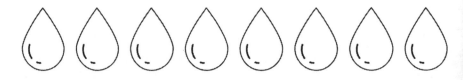

Snack 1 Time:	Symptoms/Reactions

Snack 1 Time:	Symptoms/Reactions

Snack 1 Time:	Symptoms/Reactions

Notes:

Date:_____

Breakfast Time:	Symptoms/Reactions

Lunch Time:	Symptoms/Reactions

Dinner Time:	Symptoms/Reactions

Water Intake:

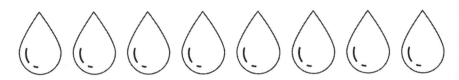

Snack 1	Time:	Symptoms/Reactions

Snack 1	Time:	Symptoms/Reactions

Snack 1	Time:	Symptoms/Reactions

Notes:

Date:_____

Breakfast Time:	Symptoms/Reactions

Lunch Time:	Symptoms/Reactions

Dinner Time:	Symptoms/Reactions

Water Intake:

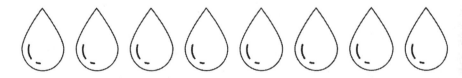

Snack 1 Time:	Symptoms/Reactions

Snack 1 Time:	Symptoms/Reactions

Snack 1 Time:	Symptoms/Reactions

Notes:

Date:_____

Breakfast Time:	Symptoms/Reactions

Lunch Time:	Symptoms/Reactions

Dinner Time:	Symptoms/Reactions

Water Intake:

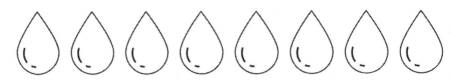

Snack 1 Time:	Symptoms/Reactions

Snack 1 Time:	Symptoms/Reactions

Snack 1 Time:	Symptoms/Reactions

Notes:

Date:_____

Breakfast	Time:	Symptoms/Reactions

Lunch	Time:	Symptoms/Reactions

Dinner	Time:	Symptoms/Reactions

Water Intake:

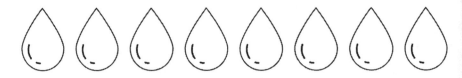

Snack 1 Time:	Symptoms/Reactions

Snack 1 Time:	Symptoms/Reactions

Snack 1 Time:	Symptoms/Reactions

Notes:

Date:_____

Breakfast Time:	Symptoms/Reactions

Lunch Time:	Symptoms/Reactions

Dinner Time:	Symptoms/Reactions

Water Intake:

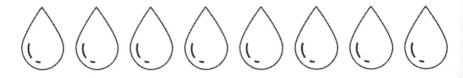

Snack 1 Time:	Symptoms/Reactions

Snack 1 Time:	Symptoms/Reactions

Snack 1 Time:	Symptoms/Reactions

Notes:

Date:_____

Breakfast Time:	Symptoms/Reactions

Lunch Time:	Symptoms/Reactions

Dinner Time:	Symptoms/Reactions

Water Intake:

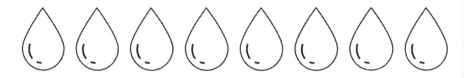

Snack 1 Time:	Symptoms/Reactions

Snack 1 Time:	Symptoms/Reactions

Snack 1 Time:	Symptoms/Reactions

Notes:

Date:_____

Breakfast Time:	Symptoms/Reactions

Lunch Time:	Symptoms/Reactions

Dinner Time:	Symptoms/Reactions

Water Intake:

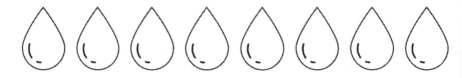

Snack 1	Time:	Symptoms/Reactions

Snack 1	Time:	Symptoms/Reactions

Snack 1	Time:	Symptoms/Reactions

Notes:

Date:_____

Breakfast Time:	Symptoms/Reactions

Lunch Time:	Symptoms/Reactions

Dinner Time:	Symptoms/Reactions

Water Intake:

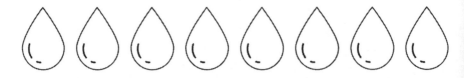

Snack 1 Time:	Symptoms/Reactions

Snack 1 Time:	Symptoms/Reactions

Snack 1 Time:	Symptoms/Reactions

Notes:

Date:_____

Breakfast Time:	Symptoms/Reactions

Lunch Time:	Symptoms/Reactions

Dinner Time:	Symptoms/Reactions

Water Intake:

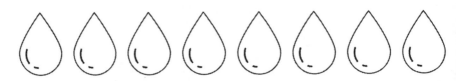

Snack 1 Time:	Symptoms/Reactions

Snack 1 Time:	Symptoms/Reactions

Snack 1 Time:	Symptoms/Reactions

Notes:

Date:_____

Breakfast	Time:	Symptoms/Reactions

Lunch	Time:	Symptoms/Reactions

Dinner	Time:	Symptoms/Reactions

Water Intake:

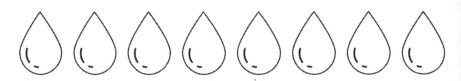

Snack 1 Time:	Symptoms/Reactions

Snack 1 Time:	Symptoms/Reactions

Snack 1 Time:	Symptoms/Reactions

Notes:

_____

_____

_____

_____

_____

Date:_____

Breakfast Time:	Symptoms/Reactions

Lunch Time:	Symptoms/Reactions

Dinner Time:	Symptoms/Reactions

Water Intake:

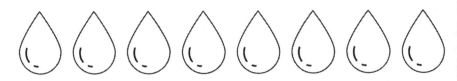

Snack 1 Time:	Symptoms/Reactions

Snack 1 Time:	Symptoms/Reactions

Snack 1 Time:	Symptoms/Reactions

Notes:

Date:_____

Breakfast Time:	Symptoms/Reactions

Lunch Time:	Symptoms/Reactions

Dinner Time:	Symptoms/Reactions

Water Intake:

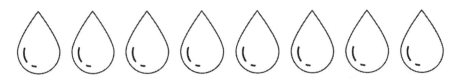

Snack 1 Time:	Symptoms/Reactions

Snack 1 Time:	Symptoms/Reactions

Snack 1 Time:	Symptoms/Reactions

Notes:

Date:_____

Breakfast Time:	Symptoms/Reactions

Lunch Time:	Symptoms/Reactions

Dinner Time:	Symptoms/Reactions

Water Intake:

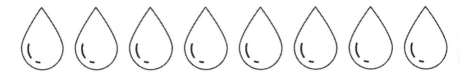

Snack 1 Time:	Symptoms/Reactions

Snack 1 Time:	Symptoms/Reactions

Snack 1 Time:	Symptoms/Reactions

Notes:

_____

_____

_____

_____

_____

Date:_____

Breakfast Time:	Symptoms/Reactions

Lunch Time:	Symptoms/Reactions

Dinner Time:	Symptoms/Reactions

Water Intake:

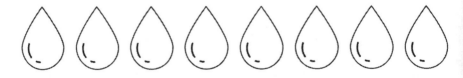

Snack 1 Time:	Symptoms/Reactions

Snack 1 Time:	Symptoms/Reactions

Snack 1 Time:	Symptoms/Reactions

Notes:

Made in the USA
Coppell, TX
22 December 2023

26815537R00053